Acupuncture Secrets

Everything you ever wanted to know
about Acupuncture and more...

Written by
Keith Baxter

What is acupuncture? It is a form of holistic healthcare that is used to prevent and treat certain diseases as well as relieve pain and anesthetize patients for surgery. Research shows that this began in China and has been practiced for more than 5,000 years.

The earliest account of this is found in the book called Nei Jing which in English means the Yellow Emperor's Classic of Internal Medicine. The contents of this book date somewhere around 200 BC. Back then, they did not use metal needles and instead used those made out of stone, moxibustion and herbs to treat a patient.

Acupuncture prevents and treats diseases by inserting very fine needles into the skin specifically at the anatomic points of the body.

The principle behind this concept is that illnesses occur because there is an imbalance in your life force otherwise known as Qi. It is believed that this flows in 14 channels in the human body known as meridians which branch out to bodily organs and functions. If there is a blockage or obstruction in any of them, this is when you succumb to a disease or an illness.

The imbalance in the Qi may go one way or the other because of Yin and Yang. The person can only be normal if there is harmony between the two which is what acupuncture is trying to achieve. This can only be restored by stimulating these acupuncture points so your Qi can be adjusted, balanced and harmonized.

Apart from using needles, practitioners also use friction, heat, impulses of electromagnetic energy and pressure to stimulate these points in order to balance the movement of energy in the body to reduce one's health.

An example of this is sonopuncture where an ultrasound device that transmits sound waves is applied to these points in the body. Some use a tuning fork and other vibration devices.

Acupressure is another example and here, the fingers are used to relive the pain. This can be used by itself or with other manual healing techniques.

Impulses of electromagnetic energy are used because our bodies generate tiny but electrical discharges which influence the function, growth and maturity of certain types of cells. By inserting the needles in these areas, it stimulates and alters the neurotransmitters in the body thus making the patient feel better after treatment. This is also sometimes used for diagnosis and testing.

According to the World Health Organization or WHO, here is a list of some illnesses where acupuncture is used. These include acute bronchitis, the common cold, cataract, toothaches, gingivitis, hiccups, ulcers, constipation, diarrhea, headache and migraine, Meniere's disease, osteoarthritis and a lot more. In the US, acupuncture is often used to treat chronic pain conditions and mind body disorders.

But acupuncture is not risk free. Hematoma may develop if the needle punctures a circulatory structure. It is also possible that pneumothorax may occur if the needle is inserted too deep. There is also the risk of HIV and hepatitis if the needle was not properly sterilized.

Now that you know what acupuncture is, you must not forget that it is merely an alternative and not a proper form of medical treatment. This means you should still be examined by a professional in the medical field who can determine the severity of your illness or disease.

With the growing acceptance of alternative medicine in Western cultures, acupuncture is quickly becoming a popular practice. More and more people today are choosing acupuncture over western medicine to treat bodily pains, relieve stress, or to promote overall health. If you are thinking about trying acupuncture but are wondering if it is safe or if it's the right treatment for you, the following information may aid you in making a more informed decision.

Description and Origin

Acupuncture is the practice of inserting fine needles into specific points in the body for therapeutic purposes. According to theory, these specific points called "acupuncture points" lie along pathways of the body along which one's vital energy is said to flow. The needles are used to promote free-flow of energy in areas of the body that circulation may have stagnated. Although acupuncture is practiced in many Asian cultures such as Japan, Tibet, and Korea the practice is commonly known to have originated in China.

Acupuncture in the Western World

One of the most debated issues between the East and the West is the use of acupuncture as a western means of medical treatment. Even though this form of medicine has been used as an effective method for over five thousand years in China, there is no concrete evidence from scientific research studies that have proven the healing properties of acupuncture.

Skeptics shrug off the positive effects of acupuncture as merely placebo effects. Believers in acupuncture, however, say that the benefits have simply not yet been proven. Believers promote that the treatment is harmless and can be used as a complement to western medicine.

Unfortunately, standards of acupuncture have not been fully approved by the FDA due to many unregulated practices that still exist such as the re-use of needles. Furthermore, acupuncture certification today is mostly a sham, used to make money on desperate patients who have not benefited from western medical treatments. The National Council Against Health Fraud has even declared acupuncture as an unproven means of treatment whose concepts of healing are primitive and false.

Should You Try It

One thing that Western science can agree upon is that there are no proven harmful effects of acupuncture. Many doctors agree that as long as a medication is not detrimental to one's health, then there is no reason why it should not be used if there are noticeable benefits. Most scientists would also state that it is simply due to a lack of research that the therapeutic properties of acupuncture have not yet been proven.

Although many forms Chinese medication remain debated concepts in Western society, there is a growing interest in these medications and perhaps as the acceptance of the practice grows, so will the discoveries about its medical properties.

More Information on Acupuncture

You can find more information about acupuncture at an acupuncture center close to you. You can easily locate nearby centers or practitioners by searching online. An appointment may be necessary as acupuncture centers are usually busy with long wait lists.

So if western medicine is not working for you and you are looking for an alternative, give some thought acupuncture. More and more people are discovering the therapeutic benefits of this ancient medicine. Acupuncture is safe and harmless, and therefore you have nothing to lose and everything to gain.

Acupuncture comes from two Latin words namely "acus" which means needle in English and "pungere" which means prick. Its history originated in China more than 2000 years ago and has evolved into various forms.

Some of the techniques of acupuncture do not even use needles anymore. Vibrating objects, ultrasound and even the fingers of the practitioner have taken some of the work to make the person feel better.

The history of acupuncture is first discussed in an ancient Chinese medical text called the "Huang Di Nei Jing" or The Yellow Emperor's Classic of Internal Medicine.

But there have been a few who are skeptic as archaeologists have found a 5,000 year old mummy in the Alps with similar acupuncture points in the body. This gives some people the idea that it was used even before the Chinese did but sine there is no written text to prove that, no one is certain and credit to this ancient practice goes back to the Chinese.

In the 6th century, this knowledge moved to Japan. In the 17th century, a man by the name of Waichi Sugiyama wanted to make this procedure painless for the patient so he developed the insertion tube, a small cylindrical tube through which the needle is inserted. Believe it or not, this technique is still being used today.

But acupuncture only reached the US in the early 80's with the establishment of a regulatory board called the National Commission for Acupuncture and Oriental Medicine. As a result, various schools have been built and those who want to become licensed acupuncturists are now able to practice their profession.

Despite that, there were a lot of people who are not yet convinced on the positive effects of alternative forms of medication. It was only in 1995 that the US Food and Drug Administration decided to classify the needles used for acupuncture as medical instruments and assured the public that they are both safe and effective.

To further promote acupuncture, the NIH or National Institute of Health in 1997 has stated that this technique is very useful in treating various health conditions.   These include ear, nose, throat, respiratory, gastrointestinal, eye, nervous system and muscular disorders. In some cases, acupuncture is able to prevent some of them from happening.

This was further strengthened by the fact that the side effects of acupuncture are much less than that of conventional drugs that are being sold by pharmaceutical companies.

So that people can avail of acupuncture, another recommendation by the NIH is for US companies to provide full coverage for certain conditions. If you do not quality, perhaps there is partial coverage which you should look up in your policy.

But despite that, more research needs to be done to see its effects on other health related problems. Some examples of these include addictions, autism, chronic low back pain, migraines and osteoarthritis of the knee.

If you look at the history of acupuncture, not much has changed since the needle technique used back then is still being used today. Even if various forms have developed through the years, one thing for sure is that it works.

In order for you to see how effective it is, you have to see a specialist who is not only qualified to treat your condition but also one is well trained.

Using needles to adjust bodily functions to optimum levels is the principle behind acupuncture. Both ancient Chinese and modern Western practitioners have used this technique to relieve many sufferers of chronic disease. Needling is a relatively safe, beneficial treatment strategy that can be used to reduce pain, improve healing, and increase general well-being. But exactly how is this procedure done and what sort of benefits can be obtained?

Procedure for Needle Puncture

There are two broad categories of acupuncture practice today, traditional Chinese medicine (TCM) and medical acupuncture. Both have their merits, so the choice is individual. The decision for most people hinges upon which philosophy appeals more to them and which technique holds the least apprehension.

In TCM, practitioners adhere to the concept of Qi, or energy flow, and the meridians in which they travel. They use longer needles and insert them deeper in order to reach the acupuncture points. Modern science has found little evidence to prove the existence of these energy channels, but this is the technique that has been used effectively for thousands of years.

In medical acupuncture, the practitioners are graduates of western medical schools. Their application of needles is not based on the traditional acupuncture points, but on anatomic data. These acupuncturists use shorter needles and the insertions are shallower. They also tend to use fewer needles and leave them inserted for shorter periods of time. Adherents to TCM feel this is a watered-down version of the real thing. Nevertheless, many patients have felt relief of symptoms through this method.

Conditions for Puncture Application

There is a broad and extensive list of ailments which can be treated with acupuncture. The conditions run the gamut from asthma to constipation, anxiety to weight loss. Most TCM practitioners believe that any health condition results from an imbalance in Qi flow, therefore amenable to needle therapy. Western acupuncturists tend to have a more limited list of indications, the most common of which is undoubtedly control of pain.

Control of pain is the most well researched of all of the indications for acupuncture. There is a definite beneficial effect for a majority of patients using this method. Migraines, premenstrual syndrome, arthritis, carpal tunnel syndrome, and neuralgias are but a few examples. The theory behind its effectiveness is also medically accepted and well researched, called the gate-control theory of pain. It states that the needles can stimulate nerves so that they block the impulses from pain triggers.

Expected Puncture Session Result

It is important to emphasize that acupuncture is used only on top of existing medical therapy. At no time should a patient discontinue medication or ignore medical instructions in favor of needle puncture. After undergoing a needle puncture regimen, the primary care physician can make an evaluation with regards to decreasing dependence on other therapies.

A course of acupuncture therapy will last anywhere from a few weeks to a few months. This depends upon the complexity of the particular medical condition. Results also vary, so it is important to have a frank discussion with the acupuncturist regarding expected results and their time frame. In general, the patient will begin to feel beneficial effects after three or four session. Certain specific conditions will actually get a little worse before improving so keeping informed is key.

In modern medicine, the use of traditional techniques with proven results has become a widely accepted practice. Acupuncture has proven its worth time and again. Modern practice guidelines make it effective, reproducible, and safe. It is a gift of healing form ancient sages that has the potential to bring relief to millions of people.

Whenever you are feeling pain and discomfort, you'd usually reach for your painkillers for relief. While they do relieve the pain, they also bring along side effects that comes with taking foreign chemicals into your body. As much as modern medicine has developed drugs that can relieve pain right off the bat, do you really think that the quick fixes you've been taking are actually good for your body? Why not try something safer and more effective like acupuncture.

What is acupuncture?

Acupuncture has surged in popularity for the last few decades as brought on by the recent health trend. Mostly known as a traditonal Chinese medical technique, acupuncture is seen as a homeopathic method of treatment. While alternative medicine does raise a lot of eyebrows for the scientifically-inclined, it does merit attention before being dismissed as a quack cure.

Basic Procedure

Basically, needles are inserted into the skin, each corresponding to one of the numerous pressure points located throughout the body. According to Traditional Chinese Medicine, by inserting a needle into the pressure point, an acupuncturist can manipulate the flow of chi or life force, thus relieving pain and gradually treating the patient. While most would say that the whole chi thing is a bunch of nonsense, science has suggested that with the needles inserted, the body's natural painkillers called endorphins are released, thus helping with pain relief.

Instruments

Modern acupuncturists nowadays use disposable fine stainless steel needles that are 0.007 to 0.020 inches in diameter which are sterilized with either ethylene oxide or by autoclave. Since they are way finer than hypodermic syringe needles, being poked by these needles are relatively painless. The upper third of the needle is covered with either a thicker bronze wire or plastic to make the needle sturdier and easier to handle. The length of the needle and how far they are inserted is all up to the acupuncturist and his practised style of acupuncture.

Example Of Treatment

If a patient has a headache, he/she is diagnosed and is treated by stimulating the sensitive points located at the webs between the thumbs and palms. In acupuncture theory, these points are connected to the face and head and can be used for treatment of headaches and other ailments involved. Needles are then carefully inserted into the skin until the patient feels a twinge, which is usually accompanied by a slight involuntary twitching of the area. During this treatment, a number of things may occur.

- Sensitivity to pain in where needles are inserted.

- A hint of nausea during treatment in case of bad headaches.

- Near-immediate headache relief.

Evolution

As an ancient method, acupuncture has crossed over into the modern age with implementations of technology and recent scientific findings. Electrical stimulation is now a common technique that is combined with acupuncture to produce more effective results. Also, acupuncturists combined this eastern technique with western methods to further enhance the treatment.

Practitioners have eventually realized that leaning towards one school of thought can't propagate progress unless they are willing to move towards the future by looking towards other horizons as well.

Reactions And Research

Not everyone is impressed with acupuncture itself. Most western medical professionals have expressed either doubt or indifference to the oriental method while others have downright driven it down into the earth with criticisms and brutal skepticism. However, recent research shows the efficacy (or lack thereof) of acupuncture, and while more research has to be done, it has been proven to actually positively affect some, but not all, forms of ailments that it claims to cure.

So as the doors open to a new age of acupuncture, give it a try when you feel the need for pain relief and you will not be disappointed. As the Chinese have used it for many centuries, so should we.

There are different types of acupuncture. Whichever you decide to use, they are designed to do the same thing and that is to relieve pain or treat certain diseases.

The first is called TCM based acupuncture. Here, it uses eight principles of complementary opposites to create harmony in the body. These include yin/yang, internal/external, excess/deficiency, hot/cold.

Next is called French energetic acupuncture. This is often used by MD acupuncturists. Meridian patterns are emphasized here particularly the yin-yang pairs of primary meridians.

Korean hand acupuncture is another as practitioners believe that the hands and feet have concentrations of qi, and that applying acupuncture needles to these areas is effective for the entire body.

There is also auricular acupuncture where it is believed that the ear is a microcosm of the body. This means that acupuncture needles are placed on certain points on the ear so it can treat certain addiction disorders.

Myofascially-based acupuncture is often utilized by physical therapists as it involves feeling the meridian lines in search of tender points before applying needles as this is where abnormal energy flows.

Japanese styles of acupuncture referred to as 'meridian therapy," tend to put more emphasis on needling technique and feeling meridians in diagnosis.

Impulses of electromagnetic energy can also be used as the body generates tiny but electrical discharges which influence the function, growth and maturity of certain types of cells. By inserting the needles in these areas, it stimulates and alters the neurotransmitters in the body thus making the patient feel better after treatment. This is also sometimes used for diagnosis and testing.

There are also other forms of acupuncture that do not use needles. For instance there is sonopuncture that uses an ultrasound device that transmits sound waves to points in the body to treat a patient. Some practitioners use a tuning fork or other vibration devices.

Acupressure is another. Here, the professional will use their hands to relieve the pain. This can be used on it sown or with other manual healing techniques.

The number of treatments you will need depends on the patient's condition. On average this could be from 10 to 5 treatments and 2 to 3 times a week. How much it will cost also varies as this could be from $40 to $150. Some insurance companies and HMO's now cover that or partially so you should check if this is included in your policy.

Anyone can try acupuncture to relieve pain or prevent one but many practitioners decline to see someone during pregnancy. But if you have already started, it is generally safe to do so until the infant is born.

Some acupuncturists may ask you to take in some herbs as part of the treatment. Since you have no idea what it can do, have this checked first by your local doctor to make sure this is safe as this could interact with the drugs you are taking causing side effects.

Which type of acupuncture should you try? That is up to you. All of them are effective so discuss this with your doctor and do some research so you know what you are getting yourself into. Each of these is painless so just relax and let the professional do the rest.

Just like conventional medicine, don't expect an improvement overnight as this takes time so just keep an open mind.

The acupuncturist is the specialist who conducts acupuncture. He or she may use needles or some other instruments depending on the type that will be used to create harmony and balance in the body.

Before this person does anything, you will first have to answer a few questions. You will then be given a physical exam to check your pulse and observe the shape, color and coating of your tongue. Other things that are checked will be the color and texture of the skin and your posture as this will give clues to your health.

Only then will you be told to lie down on a padded examining table and the needles are inserted to the skin. The difference with this kind of needle is that they twirl and jiggle each time they are pushed further into the body.

You may not feel them at all and if you do, it will only be a twitch that soon goes away. Once they are in place, this will be left there for 15 to 60 minutes that may make you feel very relaxed and sleepy that you may even doze off. Once the session is complete, the needles are removed and you will be on your way.

In some cases, acupuncture is more effective when the needles are first heated. This technique is known as 'moxibustion." Here, the acupuncturist lights a small bunch of the dried herb called moxa or mugwort and holds it above the needles. The herb, which burns slowly and gives off a little smoke and a pleasant, incense-like smell, will never directly touch your body.

Another variation is electrical acupuncture. Here, electrical wires are hooked up to the needles and a weak current runs through it which may cause no or little sensation at all.

It is also possible that herbal medications will also be prescribed by the acupuncturist for your treatment to be successful.

When looking for an acupuncturist, make sure that person is licensed. Before he or she can obtain one, they have to complete 4 years of training at an approved college of oriental medicine. In the state of California, one governing body that gives the person the title is the California Acupuncture Committee.

If they get this from another organization, a copy of their license must always be clearly displayed in the practitioner's office. One example is the National Certification Commission for Acupuncture and Oriental Medicine.

When choosing an acupuncturist, there are a few things you should ask aside from their credentials. You should know what styles of acupuncture is used as there are some techniques that do not use needles to treat a patient.

Although there are no studies which prove that one technique is better than the other, some patients are more comfortable with one type over the other.

Another question you should ask and discuss further is the length of the treatment. Patients who are suffering from a chronic illness will have to be treated over a period of months before any improvements can be seen. This will help you plan your schedule since you need to go to the clinic 2 to 3 times weekly.

The acupuncturist just like a medical doctor is there to help you get better. If you don't see any progress with this person, perhaps you should seek the help of another specialist.

There are a lot of myths with regards to acupuncture. Some of these are true; others are silly while the rest only have a half truth. As you read on, you will learn which ones are worth believing.

The first myth is that acupuncture is painful. This is not true because those who have tried it claimed they only experienced a tiny prick while others did not feel anything at all. There is no tissue damage when the needle is inserted into the skin or pulled out and only in very rare cases are there traces of bruising.

The second myth is that you can get hepatitis or AIDS from acupuncture. This is true only if the needles used are not sterilized. In the US, this will never happen because acupuncturists are required to use disposable needles thus you are not at risk from these two diseases.

Third, acupuncture is used to treat pain. This is only a half truth because this holistic technique has been proven to do other things such as stop a person's addiction, lose weight and prevent certain illnesses.

Fourth, there are some who think that Asians are the only ones that can practice acupuncture. Since 1982, there are already 50 schools all across the country that teach students about this technique and become licensed acupuncturists.

This means that anyone who has the desire to learn about this ancient practice can do so and help treat patients. Just to give you an idea, there are at least 3,000 acupuncturists now working in the US.

Fifth, medical doctors do not believe in the potential of alternative medicine. This is not true because there are more doctors these days that are open to the idea that there are other ways to help patients aside from conventional medicine. In fact, some of them even recommend an acupuncturist if they know that what they have done is not effective.

Another myth is that every patient will undergo the four needle technique. This is not true and it will only be used when the specialist feels that the energy of the patient is virtually not moving as a last resort.

The seventh myth is that it is better for a medical doctor to perform acupuncture. This is wrong because the training is much different than that taught in medical school. Students who have an acupuncturist license train for 3,000 hours before they are allowed to practice this profession. So between an acupuncturist and a medical doctor, you should go with someone who has learned about this much longer.

The eighth myth is that acupuncture is only used in third world countries. This is not true because this technique originated in China more than 2000 years ago and this has spread to developed nations in Asia such as Japan, South Korea, Singapore and Malaysia.

Here at home, acupuncture been practiced for more than 2 decades and is legal in 30 states. In fact 22 of them, license professionals after they graduate once they pass the state board examination.

Although acupuncture has been around for a very long time, there is still a need for this form of holistic healthcare which is why this is being taught in colleges and in use today. It is painless and cost efficient and a lot of studies have shown that it is effective in treating various illnesses and preventing some of them.

There are things that patients have to be aware of before, during and after surgery. The same goes for those who undergo acupuncture because in order to enhance the value of the treatment, there are some do's and don'ts that patients have to follow.

First, you should not eat a large meal before or after treatment.

You should also avoid over exercising, engaging in a sexual activity or consume alcoholic beverages 6 hours before and after treatment.

Since the acupuncture session will last from 45 minutes to 2 hours depending on how often you have to go to the clinic, you better fix your schedule so you have time to rest.

Chances are, you were consulting with a doctor prior to your visit to the acupuncturist. If there are any prescription medicines given, don't forget to take them.

You will not feel any improvement after just one or two visits with the acupuncturist. Just the same, you should write this down so you can go back to the acupuncturist on your next visit and tell him or her how you felt during the previous session. Such feedback will let the specialist know what needs to be modified in the future to help you with your problem.

The acupuncturist might give you some herbs to take as part of your treatment. Since you don't know if taking them will have any side effects with the medication you are taking, you should first consult with your doctor if it is safe to consume both.

Women who are pregnant are also advised not to undergo acupuncture treatment. However, they can engage in that once the baby is born.

How well the acupuncture treatment will go depends also on specialist who will be performing it. You have to take into account their years of experience and skill so they are able to make the correct diagnosis, finding the acupoints in the body, the angle at which the needles will be inserted and the techniques they know as there are different types of acupuncture.

This brings us to asking ourselves how to find a skill acupuncturist. For this to work, we have to do ask our doctor if they can refer anyone. It wouldn't hurt to also do some research online. After all, there are about 3,000 acupuncturists all across the country so it won't be that hard to find one.

Before you decide to have a session with them, talk to the acupuncturist to know their credentials. This will also give you the opportunity to find out how much do they charge as this can be from $45 to more than $100 per session.

You can probably ask for the name and contact number of a previous client so you can ask this person how everything went. Remember, if it doesn't work out for you, don't be afraid to find someone else who can do a better job.

The most important thing to do during the session is to relax. If you feel an itch or something, tell the acupuncturist. The same goes if you are nervous or experience a burning sensation so the specialist will take out the needles.

Now that you know the do's and don'ts of acupuncture, you should ask yourself if this form of treatment is right for you. If conventional medication doesn't work, it wouldn't hurt to see how things turn out.

Smoking is one hard habit to break. If nicotine patches and gum doesn't work, perhaps you should try something else like an alternative form of healthcare like acupuncture.

Acupuncture is an ancient practice involving the use of needles. This instrument is inserted into the skin to allow you energy or Qi to start flowing freely around your body and thus help you quit smoking.

When you go visit an acupuncturist for the first time and tell him or her that you want to quit smoking, after answering some questions, the specialist will carry out an examination of your ears and search for areas where the energy is low.

Once these spots are identified, these sharp needles are then inserted. Usually 5 needles are placed in various acupoints.

The treatment is finished after an hour and when the needles are removed, you are advised to wear ear magnets so your session continues even when you leave the clinic.   While acupuncture itself is a painless procedure, some smokers have claimed that they felt a prick or get sleepy.

Most smokers will have to come to the clinic 4 to 6 times before seeing any significant results. Just to give you an idea, one study shows that the respondents reported a decrease in the number of cravings to smoke just after one or two sessions. Seven out of 10 of the respondents were able to kick the habit after 5 or 6 sessions.

Because the number of test subjects is small, there are some who doubt the effectiveness of acupuncture.   This is because although there are positive signs with regards to the short term effects of this technique, its effects were not sustained. This is why some medical journals have stated that it is unclear what acupuncture can do in smoking cessation.

But you have to remember that acupuncture is not permanent. It merely starts something that you have to finish on your own. Some smokers who go 2 or 3 times a week to the clinic will need to come back for follow up sessions in the future.

At the same time, you have to find ways to prevent yourself from picking up a cigarette. You can do this by staying away from people who smoke since you will be tempted to ask for a stick. You can create your own personal mantra which you repeat to yourself every time you have an urge.

Remember that this craving is only short term and will last only for a few minutes. You have worked so hard to leave this behind so stick to the path and stay smoke free.

Acupuncture treatment for smokers should only be done by a license professional. You can do some research online to find out if they are accredited by the National Commission for Acupuncture and Oriental Medicine, ask how long they have been in the profession, find out how many smokers they have helped and how much will they charge.

Once you have found one, you have to commit yourself to the program because both you and the acupuncturist have to work together to give up this habit.

Acupuncture can help smokers in the same way that it has helped addicts and alcoholics quit their addictions. You just have to try it even if you may not believe in it.

Studies have shown that there is an increase in the number of children that have been diagnosed with autism. Until now, doctors have not yet found a cure to this illness which is why some parents want to experiment with alternative forms of treatment and one example is acupuncture.

Acupuncture is a holistic approach in treating and preventing certain diseases. Its main tool are very thin needles that are inserted to targeted points in the body. The body has about 400 of them linked through a system known as meridians or pathways. Once these are stimulated, these are supposed to create balance in the body.

Autism on the other hand is a brain disorder that is long term. This disease is characterized by deficits in language, social communication and cognition. Children who are diagnosed with this illness may also suffer from secondary problems such as aggression, irritability, stereotypes, hyperactivity, negativism, volatile emotions, temper tantrums, short attention span and obsessive-compulsive behavior.

Preliminary studies have shown that acupuncture may provide symptomatic relief to children suffering from autism. Although difficult at first, it is believed that it is rewarding in the long run. This is because while conventional therapy and treatment requires that the child stay still, acupuncture doesn't. Some say it's a quick prick at the vital points in the body.

A group of children in the US participated in a test to see how effective acupuncture is among children. There are 22 respondents and each of them was given the treatment once every other day for four months.

After the treatment 20 out of the 22 respondents showed remarkable improvement. In fact 2 of them has cerebral blood flow.   The only thing that did not change prior to treatment and after was the blood flow between the left and right cerebrum as it showed no differences.

Aside from traditional acupuncture to help children with autism, a preliminary study in Hong Kong is trying to see if tongue acupuncture can produce better results.

Results have showed that of 30 respondents in the test, majority showed functional improvement of various degrees depending on the age and severity of their disabilities. Some improvement was noticeable within a few TAC sessions, especially for drooling, spasticity (scissoring or tiptoeing), ataxia, and poor balance in walking. Functional improvement was noted after one to two courses of TAC. Most children tolerated TAC well, with only occasional pain and minor bleeding in some patients.

The reason why tongue acupuncture is being experimented with is because there is a connection between the tongue and the heart through the meridians that spread to all the organs in the body. It is believed that the points on the tongue can influence the state of the other body organs thus giving relief to the one suffering from autism.

But many believe that acupuncture alone cannot help autism sufferers. It has to be combined with other things like maintaining a certain diet to help improve one's mood and communication schools. Although it is only short term, it is better than nothing until a cure is found.

When will the cure be found? Only time can tell as there are many other questions that have to be answered in order for doctors to further understand neurological disabilities. Doctors who are conducting research believe that an interdisciplinary approach is needed given that acupuncture has shown positive results in helping children with autism.

Today's world can fill the very busy individual with a lot of stress. Without some way of removing this stress from your system, you're placing yourself in danger from a lot of stress-related diseases. You might suffer from insomnia or headaches or very serious heart diseases.

You could take anti-stress pills to help you relax but, like me, you might also be worried about the side effects these pills could have. The good news is that you could try acupuncture at least once to see if it could help you manage the stress. It certainly couldn't hurt to try acupuncture if all you're after is stress relief.

If you find it doesn't work for you, then you can just easily stop taking acupuncture treatments. If it works, though, then you can say you've found a good treatment for stress that doesn't rely on those dangerous chemicals and pills.

How does sticking needles into your body help manage the stress?

In traditional Chinese medicine, much of the treatments depend on an understanding of the balance in our bodies and its internal organs. The sicknesses we sometimes develop are seen to be caused by imbalances in our lifestyles and environment. Stress is also affected by this imbalance. That is why when there is something wrong with your body, you'd typically have less of an ability to deal with stress. You'd get more irritable and find it really to difficult to relax.

By sticking these very thin needles past the surface of our skin, the acupuncturist stimulates nerves in our body. These nerves send signals to our brain and scientists believe that the brain then releases its natural painkillers into our system. This immediately causes a feeling of relaxation for many people.

The needles could also help your body by stimulating its circulation. With the circulation between the organs of the body improved, a lot of the body's wastes could be cleansed properly. Your organs would also receive the full benefit of the oxygen from your lungs making its way into the cells of your body without any blockages. This makes your organs much healthier and leaves you feeling much better in the long term as well.

You can think of a session with the acupuncturist as very much like massage therapy. A good massage would help give you a very relaxing sleep that night and an acupuncturist could help you with your sleep as well. You might immediately start to feel drowsy as soon as the right nerves are stimulated by the acupuncturist's needles.

You might be asking yourself how you'd be able to relax if you're suffering from the pain of the needles attached to your body. What you might not realize is that because of the thinness of the needles, you would hardly feel anything. The most that many people claim they feel is a kind of tingling feeling where the needles are. And that is actually a sign that the process is working,

Acupuncture is a practice that helps you use your bodies' own ability to manage stress properly.

This leaves you healthier, and more importantly, prevents any of the serious diseases that could come from unbalanced, stressful lifestyles.

It might not be something to replace regular trips to the doctor but with its many possible benefits, acupuncture might be worth trying out very soon.

Acupuncture can help treat migraines. This was discovered after a comparative study was done with conventional medical care. In some cases, it even prevents it from happening which helps improve the quality of life for the patient.

To understand how acupuncture helps migraine sufferers, you have to understand that in traditional Chinese medicine, it is believed that an imbalance in the flow of blood and energy causes this to happen.

In order to treat it, the specialist must relieve the tension by inserting needles into the body to improve the blood flow to the brain thus reducing the pain experienced during an attack.

The needles used helps the body balance the serotonin levels since it is a neurotransmitter that affects blood vessels and has a role to play in migraines.   In fact the more frequent these sessions are the better. It may even come to a point where the specific point of contact is no longer needed but the general stimulation itself.

The end result of undergoing acupuncture is amazing. If you experience 15 to 20 days of agonizing pain, this may be count down to only 8 days. You won't even need to use that much medication anymore as before.

For those who are working, this is good so that they are not absent from work that much and there won't be that much deductions in their salary.

But how well acupuncture does for one patient may vary with another. This depends on the condition of the attack and the individual.

The best part about acupuncture is that there are no side effects and it is painless. Skillful professionals can do this so you don't suffer from hematoma or pneumothorax. Another disease is potentially dangerous is HIV or hepatitis which can be prevented of course as long as the needles used are properly sterilized. It will be much better if the person uses disposable needles.

Acupuncture has been practiced in the United States for more than 2 decades. Although tests have shown how effective it can be to treat chronic conditions and certain addictions, more studies need to be done to see where else it can be useful.

Although one test has proven that acupuncture can help migraines, other tests will also have to be done to prove if this is true. Until such time that other results are published, patients will have to rely on conventional medicine that is prescribed by a doctor.

But you don't have to wait for the results to come out. If you think it is worth a try, go for it. Just ask for a referral from your doctor as there are many practitioners who have accepted the fact that alternative forms of medicine can also help a patient.

You can also find someone online. You can be sure they are certified if they are recognized by the National Certification Commission for Acupuncture and Oriental Medicine.

Aside from that, you should also make some lifestyle changes as there are trigger factors that have been known to cause migraines. Stress is number one on the list so you get enough rest and exercise as well as a balanced diet.

Patients who are suffering from migraine should also check if acupuncture is covered by their HMO. Most insurance providers and HMO's these days cover all or part of the cost but there are restrictions so you should check what is covered by your policy.

In a generation when physical fitness is given topmost attention, people are always on the lookout for the newest and most effective means for weight loss. Acupuncture, the method of inserting thin, filiform needles on certain points in an individual's body, has been found to be one effectual method for losing weight.

Not many people may find the idea of being inserted by needles quite comforting in their quest for weight control. However, this ancient Chinese alternative treatment seeks to deliver a control mechanism, enabling the patient to manage hunger cravings more successfully in the long run.

The Skinny on Acupuncture Weight Loss

It has been found that weight gain is directly related to emotions.   Other than physical hunger, people reach for a huge chocolate bar or a big platter of burger and fries because of the sense of comfort derived from food and eating. More often than not, excessive weight gain is an emotional issue, rather than a mere physical one. You may not realize it, but you tend to take in more food whenever you"re stressed, upset, or pressured.

In Acupuncture, there are specific spots on the body being targeted by the hair-like needles. These spots are linked to certain areas in the body and by stimulating these spots; the patient will achieve a greater sense of inner balance. As these points are inserted by the needles, certain hormones are released throughout the body. These substances work by helping you manage hunger and efficiently control the impulse to overeat.

How Acupuncture Induces Weight Loss

Most acupuncturists will target the spots behind the ear when it comes to promoting weight loss. When these points behind the ear are stimulated, endorphins are released in large doses. Endorphins are called the feel-good hormones, and these are also often referred to as natural pain and fever relievers. The release of endorphins is what makes you feel better after an increased level of physical activity, as in the case of a good workout.

These bodily compounds allow the patient to experience better relaxation, thus considerably alleviating stress. There is a greater possibility of enhanced weight loss when the patient has already achieved emotional wellness. Endorphins are also released whenever the body experiences low levels of bodily pain, thus their moniker as a natural pain reliever.

Patients of acupuncture typically experience very minimal or no pain at all, however most of the points are located near nerve endings and muscle tissues. As the needles are embedded in the body, signals are sent to the brain thus promoting the release of endorphins from the pituitary gland.

There are also other points in the body that serve as gateways for better weight management. One of these placements promotes a decrease in an individual's appetite, while another has the ability to reduce water retention in the body. The acupuncturist may choose a multi-targeted approach, depending on the requirements of the patient.

Consulting with a Professional Acupuncturist

There are a number of acupuncture practitioners in existence nowadays, offering a host of services. If you are considering this form treatment for your weight management, make sure that you settle with no less than a trained and professional acupuncturist. A poorly trained acupuncturist may not be able to pinpoint the specific meridian points and worse, may cause unnecessary bodily pain and discomfort.

Moreover, your acupuncturist may require an herbal supplement for your treatment, to encourage a longer-term effect. Your sessions need not be maintained for an extensive period; however you may be required to visit your acupuncturist during the entire course of the sessions.

There are other means for losing weight successfully, and this does not include crash dieting and strenuous work outs. If carried out by trained professionals, acupuncture can be the answer for effective weight management. While it is far from being a cure-all, it may just be the right weight loss solution for you.

The foundation of acupuncture rests on the relevance of an individual's chi in maintaining bodily and mental health. It is believed that chi is present in every living creature, and flows through specific pathways in the body. Health problems arise when the flow of chi on the body is blocked. As a result, a person may feel persistent headaches, muscle pain, fever, weakness, or in the worst case, becomes afflicted with more serious health conditions.

A Deeper Explanation of Acupuncture

Acupuncture has its origins in ancient Chinese philosophy and practice. More than ten thousand years ago, during the Old Stone Age of China, stones were fashioned into knives for medical purposes. After several years, during the New Stone Age, these stones were eventually made into needles intended for the same therapeutic end. These accounts are further evidenced by unearthed stone needles found to be of the same types used during the New Stone Age.

There are basically 14 pathways throughout the body where chi flows continuously. These are called the meridian points. In order for chi to course through the body unobstructed, there has to be a balance between the strengths of yin and yang. In ancient Chinese philosophy, yin and yang represent the forces of the universe- yin is for feminine, while yang is for masculine. Every single thing in the universe is believed to contain both yin and yang for harmony.

When the yin and yang are not balanced, chi cannot stream through the body liberally. Therefore, the meridian points through which chi courses through need to be stimulated. This is done by the insertion of hair-thin, disposable needles in specific areas on a person's body to induce bodily harmony and bring about healing.

A certified and trained acupuncturist will be able to carry out an excellent therapy session for the patient. Trainings for acupuncturists are given in order for them to obtain their licenses. A poor practitioner may not be proficient enough with the practice and could end up jeopardizing the results of the entire procedure. Nowadays, it is wise to verify on a practitioner's credentials to ensure a safe and effective acupuncture treatment.

What This Ancient Method Does

One of the foremost effects of acupuncture on the body is relaxation. Stress is frequently pinpointed as the main precursor for a host of physical ailments. There are particular points all over the body that direct the flow of harmony and relaxation and when these are enthused, the patient becomes more at ease.

Another positive effect of this alternative therapy is increased pain control. During a session, a patient will usually feel very minimal pain as the thin needles are being inserted gradually. However, the needles are deliberately placed in varying depths, depending on the health requirements of the patient. When the needles reach the right depth, the patient will feel deeper pain, although the entire procedure is not necessarily painful.

It is also recommended for relief from chemotherapy fatigue as well as chemotherapy-related nausea. It has also been found to be largely effective for back pains, migraines, menstrual cramps, and as a pain controller for patients after undergoing surgical operations.

Variations of Conventional Acupuncture

Auriculotherapy or ear acupuncture is one of the variations of conventional acupuncture. In this practice, it is believed that the ear provides a map for all the major bodily organs. A specific area or point on the ear corresponds to a particular organ, such as the heart, kidneys, or liver. Thus, the needles are placed in particular points around the ear and on the ear cartilage.

Staplepuncture is a method used in smoking cessation, wherein staples are placed for a certain period anywhere on the ear area to provide stimulation.

Indeed there is growing evidence that this traditional Oriental practice can rival any modern forms of treatment. If you are one of the many people who are looking for a widely recognized and time honored therapeutic practice, acupuncture may just be the alternative treatment for you.

Have you ever had an uncontrollable urge to be pierced by a dozen needles? This is the image most people get when someone mentions the word "acupuncture". It comes as no surprise that most view this technique with suspicion, even downright horror. The fact is, however, that this relatively painless ancient Chinese technique has helped relieve the symptoms of millions of people. Properly used, it can help in the management of many medical conditions including chronic pain and fatigue.

How does needle puncture work?

Practitioners of Chinese traditional medicine believe in energy flows. This energy, called Qi, circulates around the body using pathways called meridians. Meridians run very close to the surface of the skin in certain areas and can be accessed by needles. Much like plumbing, these pipes can get blocked or go the wrong way, causing health problems. The insertion of needles at these points is aimed to help loosen blocks and normalize flow.

It sounds like a made-up explanation with no basis in reality, but there are numerous scientific studies which support the effects of acupuncture. Although the exact scientific basis is still unknown, recent theories seem to suggest involvement of complicated neurochemical effects in the brain, nerve to spinal cord impulse modulation, and microscopic connective tissue changes. What risks and side effects are of concern?

The use of things not completely understood for the treatment of medical conditions is nothing new. Penicillin and aspirin were used for decades solely on the basis of their beneficial effects, without doctors knowing exactly how they worked. Results are what are truly important. However, it is equally important is to ensure that the technique is used safely.

Like other strategies used in treating health conditions, acupuncture may have some side effects. Medications have side effects and allergic reactions, surgeries have risk of infection and complications. For needle puncture, there is a risk of injury, rare infections, minor bleeding, small bruises, and some dizziness.

You can minimize the possible side effects by choosing a licensed acupuncturist. Most countries either have government licensing in place or have professional organizations with very strict rules and regulations.

How do treatments go?

An acupuncturist will do an initial evaluation of your medical history and your body's current state. Multiple pressure points are palpated, and a regimen of treatment is formulated. Most courses involve a series of 10 to 20 treatment sessions, each lasting 30 to 90 minutes. Needles will be carefully placed at the required points and kept in place for some time. Most patients report a feeling of mild sensation at the site of the puncture, but no real pain.

Right after each acupuncture session, you will feel a bit tired and may need to rest. Some people feel an increase in their energy levels. The response to acupuncture is very individual. In some cases there is immediate relief of symptoms. For some patients, the beneficial effects may only be noticed after undergoing a few sessions. Do not be alarmed and keep your acupuncturist updated on what you are feeling to ensure everything is going as expected.

You need never fear the thought of needles ever again. Acupuncture is a beneficial treatment with a long history of effectiveness. It is used to complement current medical therapy and should not replace currently existing medications or treatments.

The safe application of this once exclusively Chinese therapy can now be experienced by chronic disease sufferers worldwide.

If you want to pursue a career in acupuncture, you need to obtain a degree and become a licensed professional.

This can easily be accomplished in three years of schooling from an accredited alternative medicine school which prepares students in the various acupuncture techniques to treat illnesses resulting from allergies, occupational stress, emphysema, gastrointestinal stress, arthritis, headaches, depression, and hypertension to name a few.

Students who enroll in such courses will be taught through demonstration, discussion and hands on application.

Part of the curriculum will also include basic courses in traditional medicine covering subjects such as anatomy, biosciences, medical terminology, herbal medicine, moxibustion, and acupressure. In some schools, they may require students to also learn about nutrition and various kinds of research.

Once they graduate, they may start in an entry level position earning $40,000 or more which will soon double or triple after years of experience and working themselves up the ladder.

If you want to look for a school that offers acupuncture degrees, it is best to go online and see which one has the best program that suits your requirements.

You won't have a hard time looking for one as the number of institutions which teach students about acupuncture have gone up at a rapid rate since 1982 when the Accreditation Commission for Acupuncture and Oriental Medicine (ACAOM) and the Council of Colleges of Acupuncture and Oriental Medicine (CCAOM) were established.

To date there are about 50 colleges and a few also offer a master's degree in Oriental Medicine and Acupuncture.

So what are you waiting for? If you think you have what it takes to be an acupuncturist, then go ahead and just do it.

It doesn't matter if you are still in high school or if you are already working because a shift in your career could let you achieve your true calling.

The best way to start though is to talk with an acupuncturist about what it takes to become one so he or she will be able to give you an idea of what happens in the job.

If you haven't picked a school, talk to students about the curriculum so you get your money" s worth should you decide to attend this college.

A lot of people are unaware that acupuncture is not yet legal in every state. You can find work or start your own practice in California, New York, Texas, Hawaii and Oregon with 8 more states that are still pending legislation.

We mentioned that you have to study in a school certified by the Council of Colleges of Acupuncture and Oriental Medicine (CCAOM). One more hurdle you have to face before getting your license is passing an exam given by them except in the state of California which has its own regulating body and board certification exam in order for you to practice your profession.

An acupuncturist degree is just the first step in becoming your own boss. To become a master, you have to learn everything there is to know as a student so those who entrust themselves to you in the future will not have any problems.

As more people are opening their minds to this practice, people should know that getting an acupuncture degree will not replace traditional medicine since there are limits to what it can do for the patient. It is merely a form of holistic healthcare that works hand in hand with science to help the person deal with an illness.

If, like me, you have quite a fear of needles and injections, then acupuncture, that practice of sticking needles onto different parts of your body to cure sicknesses might seem scary at first.

However, if you've been long been suffering from some problems like headaches or chronic pains and your regular visits to the doctor don't seem to be helping you, then why not consider a trip to an acupuncture specialist? After all, who hasn't heard of somebody's aunt somewhere suffering from arthritis and trying out everything that the doctors recommended all to no avail, only to finally be cured by a really good acupuncturist?

Perhaps you were wondering if it could actually work for you. You might feel a bit skeptical since traditional Chinese medicine doesn't immediately coincide with theories in modern Western medicine. In fact, the use of needles to cure people was discovered thousands of years ago in China long before microscopes or x-ray machines were invented or before bacteria and germs were discovered.

When you think about it, that might be something that the practice has going for it. If it has existed already for thousands of years and is still being practiced by millions up to now, then it must have worked already for quite a number of people.

What typically happens when you go to an acupuncturist?

When you go to an acupuncturist, you would typically first be asked about your medical history, how you're feeling and any symptoms of sicknesses you might have. The specialist would observe features of your face, including your tongue. According to specialists, your tongue is a good indicator of the health of your internal organs. The acupuncturist would listen to sounds that your body makes like the sounds coming from your lungs. How your body smells could also be an indicator of your overall health for the acupuncturist's diagnosis.

Based on what the acupuncturist finds out about your sickness, he or she would then formulate the treatment that your body needs. With traditional Chinese medicine, sicknesses are seen as a kind of imbalance and loss of harmony between your bodies' organs. You can consider the use of needles on your body as just a way to push your body and its organs back into balance.

The specialist would begin inserting very thin needles into the right places in your body. To many people, inserting these needles doesn't really hurt. After all, an acupuncturist's needles are usually much thinner than the needles that are used for injections. Many have claimed that inserting these needles actually calms them down and relaxes them.

How does the use of these needles help you?

A lot of problems have been claimed to have been alleviated through this practice. These include headaches, the common cold, arthritis, back pains, asthma and even infertility.

Even though acupuncture isn't part of Western medicine, Western medicine experts have studied it extensively. Some theories as to why it works involve acupuncture perhaps stimulating the brain's release of the body's natural painkillers. Acupuncture could also stimulate proper circulation in the human body.

Western medicine is still studying acupuncture and trying to find out how to best integrate it with practices in Western medicine. That is why, along with Western medicine and trips to the doctor, one could certainly try acupuncture.

It couldn't hurt and it might actually be the one to finally relieve you of a lot of your body's aches and pains and even make you healthier.

There are a lot of people who are overweight. For those who are obese, perhaps surgery is the best option but for those who can't, they can try to see if acupuncture can help take out the excess weight.

Acupuncture is a form of holistic healthcare that uses needles to help treat a patient.   Unlike the cartoon where the balloon will pop and all the air will go out, the needles that are inserted into the vital points will stimulate the body to release endorphins thus helping the person control their appetite.

But before needles are inserted, the specialist will first ask the patient some questions and perform an examination. This is needed to understand the main cause for the person to be overweight.

Part of examination is to help the acupuncturist figure out where the needles will be inserted. Your pulse will give the person an idea on your general state of energy and the general health of your stomach.

You will also have to open your mouth and show your tongue to check for cracks, peelings or puffiness on the stomach area as this provides clues to why you are overweight.

Once he or she knows the reason, this is the time that the needles are inserted into different parts of the body. One way is called the multi-targeted approach which is designed to lower the body's weight by increasing the output of the pituitary gland.

The areas where the needles will be inserted will be in the ear and in two of three body points. These areas could also include the mouth, the stomach, the lung, the endocrine, the spleen, kidney or thyroid.

During the initial treatment, the "Four Gate" points would be used to circulate energy throughout the entire body. It is also possible that electro simulation will also be done to increase endorphin release and stimulate metabolism.

These needles will be kept in place for 30 to 45 minutes depending on how much support is needed. These are then removed and replaced with ear tacs with adhesives to make sure they are in the same spot as the needles.

These ear tacs work by applying mild pressure whenever he or she feels hungry. It causes a mild endorphin release and helps the patient relax making it possible to use their willpower and resist the temptation to eat.

The patient will also have to reduce cravings on certain food by cutting down the intake. Some studies suggest that this can also lower insulin levels or lipid levels in the blood.

The best part about acupuncture is that there are no harmful side effects and no chance for an addiction to occur. The patient will have to come back for regular treatment and have to pay attention to one's diet and exercise regularly as needles can only do so much to control one's weight.

The number of treatments for someone who is overweight varies depending on how many pounds they want to lose, the speed at which they want to lose it and their commitment to sticking to the plan.

The average patient on the other hand who wants to lose 5 to 10 pounds will have to come for treatment every three days or twice a week then once this is attained, once every two weeks. It is up to the person until when the treatment will be done which shows that acupuncture can help you lose weight.

Holistic healthcare by definition is being able to cure an illness through the use alternative means. This means no medication is given to the patient and an instrument like a bunch of needles could do the trick.

Acupuncture has been around for than 2000 years. It is only recently that this holistic form of healthcare has reached the US. Studies have shown that it can treat minor problems and prevent some from happening.

The needles used in acupuncture are very thin but thicker than the human hair. This makes it smaller than those used on hypodermic needles.

Most patients that undergo acupuncture will not feel any significant change after one session which is why a few sessions are needed. Best of all, it is painless so your body will not feel sore afterwards.   Several studies have been conducted about acupuncture and there have been positive results. For instance in the UK, 400 participants who were suffering from migraines claimed they felt better after 3 months worth of sessions.

In the US, acupuncture has also proven to be effective in helping people deal with arthritis because the needles help the body fight against this chronic illness that is much cheaper and more effective than conventional medicine.

Acupuncture can do more than just helping patients deal with arthritis or migraine. Clinical tests have shown that it can help obese people lose weight and those who are suffering from insomnia.

In some countries, acupuncture has even been used to replace chemical anesthesia prior to surgery as there are some patients who are not able to tolerate regular anesthesia.

Another field which acupuncture has proven to be effective is helping patients deal with their addictions such as alcohol, drugs and smoking. One study of smokers revealed that the average patient will cut down by half the number of cigarettes they consume after just one treatment. Just imagine the potential after a few more sessions!

This has resulted in the establishment of clinics nationwide that only use acupuncture as the means of rehabilitation.

Acupuncturists in the US charge from $75 to $150 per session. This usually gets lower in the succeeding treatments.   The person will probably have to undergo 10 to 15 treatments 2 to 3 times a week but this really depends on the condition of the patient.   Before you go to one, you should check if this is covered by your insurance. If it isn't, perhaps you should suggest that it should be included as it is much cheaper than having to undergo surgery.

Although there are risks if you decide to go undergo acupuncture, these can be avoided as long as the one doing it is a licensed professional who makes sure that the needles used are sterilized before they are inserted into the body.

These days, a lot of people in the medical field have accepted the fact that alternative medicine such as this can also help the patient which is why they may refer someone when it is needed.

So, if you are tired of experiencing the side effects of conventional medicine and want to try a holistic form of healthcare, why don't you see what acupuncture can do for you? It is painless and cost effective. In fact, it is just one of many you can try to help treat a chronic condition.

Acupuncture is already a renowned method used in treating smoking addiction. An alternative medicine believed to have originated as far as 3000 BC in ancient China, this treatment is now being widely utilized for various medicinal and therapeutic purposes. It has been found furthermore to successfully treat drug dependence and chronic smoking addiction.

There are several smoking cessation medications and therapies available presently. However acupuncture is a recommended alternative procedure, especially where conventional therapies have already failed. The strategic insertion of needles in various parts of the body aims to treat the condition in a more profound and emotional level. A smoker needs to free himself from the physiological and psychological addiction of smoking, thus necessitating a more holistic treatment.

How It Stops the Addiction

The placement of needles is usually located behind the ear, or on the ear cartilage. This is where the calming effect takes place, curbing the patient's cravings for more cigarettes. People who have a smoking habit are bound to take up the nicotine stick more often whenever they feel stressed, bored, or depressed. Needles are also often inserted on the hand and wrists to promote a steadier flow of bodily energy. The feeling of relaxation will help an individual think twice about lighting a cigarette again.

Furthermore, this treatment has been found to help an individual deal with the withdrawal symptoms better.   This alternative medicine promotes better tolerance to pain and discomfort during smoking cessation. Withdrawal symptoms can range from mild to severe and may involve nausea, palpitations, and dizziness. Oftentimes, these same conditions will propel an individual back to his smoking tendencies sooner than later.

Nicotine is the addictive and toxic substance present in a cigarette. This is the same substance that makes quitting a big challenge for most smokers. The nicotine that you get from smoking will attach itself to the pleasure areas in the brain, making it hard for you to stop. Without a steady stream of this substance, a smoker will tend to feel depressed and uncomfortable.

People who have undergone acupuncture treatment reported that they no longer find cigarettes as tempting or as satisfying. Oftentimes, smoking would leave an awful taste in their mouths prompting them to stop their habit for once. Some patients would even resort to eating mints or lozenges to clear to get rid of the terrible aftertaste.

According to skilled practitioners, approximately 7 out of 10 smokers will successfully extricate themselves from their smoking habit after 2 or 3 weeks. While the others are unable to quit totally, these smokers will be able to cut down on their cigarette consumption quite significantly.

Treatment from Acupuncture Experts

It is very essential for a patient to consult with a skilled acupuncturist. A more personalized service will be provided by an expert, as well as added counseling for the patient. Moreover, an acupuncturist may prescribe herbal supplements to aid the patient in quitting efforts.

During treatment, filiform needles are inserted into specific points on the ear cartilage, as well as the hands and wrists. Normal procedures last for about 30 minutes. Body acupuncture can be used in combination with the ear and wrist needle placements. An acupuncturist may also utilize a mild electric current, to enhance the effect of the needles through the body.

The greatest advantage of this ancient Oriental procedure is the absence of side-effects during and after treatment. Unlike smoking cessation medications and nicotine replacement therapy products, acupuncture does not employ chemically manufactured substances. There is also no risk of weight gain during therapy. In conjunction with helping a patient quit smoking, it can also curb appetite, thus reducing food cravings.

If you have tried several methods in smoking cessation to no avail, perhaps it is high time you consider the alternative method that is acupuncture. With the right practitioner and the right frame of mind, there is no reason why you won't be nicotine-free before long.

Since 1982, acupuncture has found its way to the US. There are currently 50 schools that teach it and 3,000 licensed practitioners all over the country. Do you think you can be a licensed professional? Here are a few things to help you look for a good acupuncture school.

You should now that the 50 schools mentioned are all accredited by the National Commission for Acupuncture and Oriental Medicine.   It is recognized by the Department of Education and some of these schools even have a masters program.

Most of these schools can be found online so you can give them a call and ask certain questions about the school. You can find out the cost of tuition, the teacher student ratio, if the school offers consultation services to students and the alumni and if they have an extensive library which focuses on traditional Chinese medicine.

Should there be a school near where you live, you should probably take it so you don't have to worry about boarding and lodging as this is just added cost to this long term investment.

If you like the school but cannot afford the cost of tuition, find out if they offer scholarships or if they have a grant in aid program. If there are none, then check with the federal government because they should have one and they will give it to deserving students who plan to enroll in a school accredited by the National Commission for Acupuncture and Oriental Medicine.

Some states do not require you to get a license once you graduate from the program. However, if you plan to practice this elsewhere, you should prepare yourself for the state board exam as this is a requirement.

The lists of subjects you will be learning in school include anatomy, body therapy, massage therapy and the other sciences. Training will be done also in a clinical setting so you are able to put theory into practice but this will only happen in your third year.

While some schools will let you finish a program in three years, there are those that can be completed after five.

Lately, acupuncture school has also gone down the digital path by offering cyber distance programs for those who cannot go to school. Some of these offer CEU's or continuing education units to advance programs.

These courses can be chosen on the basis of modules or on an hourly basis. The course material covers the history, theory and techniques of acupuncture. Courses that offer tools such as acupuncture DVD and video are ideal for acupuncturists or students of acupuncture to improve their clinical expertise.

Once you graduate from acupuncture school, some will open their own practice while others will first work for a clinic. Those who decide to be employed will work with other professionals that may include naturopaths, chiropractors and other specialists that are also into Oriental Medicine.

The average acupuncturist makes about $45,000 a year but this can change in the years to follow as they add years or experience under their belt. This just goes to show that if you work hard, you too will make a fortune. Just make sure that you do this properly for each patient because one mistake could make this all go away.

Are you an individual who suffers from allergies?   If so, you may be looking for ways to seek relief.   Most individuals turn to over-the-counter medications.   While these medications do work, in most cases, there are many individuals who are concerned with exactly what it is they are putting into their bodies.   If you are one of those individuals, you will want to continue reading on.   Below, a number of natural allergy remedies are highlighted below.   In addition to being considered natural allergy remedies, many are also known as home remedies for allergies.

One natural allergy remedy that comes highly rated and recommended is that of apple cider vinegar.   Often times, the only complaint that most have with apple cider vinegar is the taste.   However, it is not only known as a natural remedy to treat allergies.   Many also use it to assist with weight loss, high blood pressure, and high cholesterol.   Most individuals using apple cider vinegar to treat allergies recommend taking two tablespoons a day.   Mixing it with juice or water is also advised, which can assist with taste issues.

Red clover is another natural allergy remedy.   What is nice about using red clover to treat your allergy symptoms is all of the options that you have, as red clover is available in a wide range of formats.   With that being said, most allergy sufferers recommend red clover tea.   Red clover wine and red clover herbal supplements, which come in the format of pills, are also available for sale both on and offline.

Carefully choosing the foods in which you consume is another natural way to reduce or treat the symptoms of allergies.   Lime squeezed into water has been known to assist those with allergies.   Vegetable juices and bananas also come highly rated and recommended.

Acupuncture is also an ideal way to treat and relieve the symptoms of allergies.   According to WebMD, a trusted medical website, acupuncture helped to reduce all allergy symptoms in a study performed on twenty-six patients.   If you are interested in giving acupuncture a try, consider contacting your local health spas, as many offer alternative healing approaches.   If acupuncture is not a service offered, you should be provided with contact information for another local practitioner.

In addition to the above mentioned natural allergy remedies, there are also steps that you can take to prevent the onset of allergies or steps that you can take to reduce these symptoms.   Most of these helpful tips can still be considered natural allergy remedies, but in a different sense.   Also, these additional tips, a few of which are outlined below, are for just about anyone suffering from allergies, as they are affordable and easy to implement.

 For pet allergies, stay a safe distance away from pets.   With that said, if you are a pet owner who cannot bear to part with your beloved pets, be sure to keep them out of your bedroom, as this is where you spend most of your time.

Since mold is a common trigger factor for allergies, it is important to take steps to remove mold from your home or prevent it from growing.   Limiting the humidity in your home is a great way to reduce or completely prevent mold growth.   Use a bathroom fan or open a bathroom window when taking a shower, to reduce mold growth in the bathroom.   If you already have mold in your home, contact a professional to inquire about a mold removal.   Until that time comes, be sure to avoid areas in your home where mold is present.

The above mentioned natural allergy remedies are just a few of the many that allergy sufferers recommend, but they are a few of the most popular approaches taken.   As a reminder, it is important to remember that natural remedies and home remedies work differently on different individuals.   If you do not see the success that you had hoped for, not all hope is lost, as there should be another natural allergy remedy out there that can provide you with relief.

Looking beautiful both inside and out is something we all want to achieve. Since your face is ridden with emotion and hormonal issues, you have to take care of it. Fortunately, there is a technique that can do that using painless mini needles and this is better known as facial acupuncture.

Facial acupuncture is a painless procedure that renews not only the face but the body as well. This is because it can erase lines and eye bags making you look younger. At the same time, it can also help clear up pimples and acne.

For this to work, fine needles are placed in acupuncture points on the eyes, face and neck to stimulate the person's natural energies.   As a result, this also improves your facial color.

Anyone can try facial acupuncture because it is painless and it has proven to reverse the signs of aging. However, if you are pregnant, suffer from the colds or flu, have acute herpes or an allergic reaction, it is best to wait until this has passed.

But before anyone can try facial acupuncture, they first have to be evaluated by the acupuncturist. This person will evaluate your age, lifestyle and diet. If everything looks good, then you will probably do an average of about 12 to 15 treatments. More could be done if your skin tends to sag, manifest jowls or have droopy eyes.

Facial acupuncture treatment needs to be done twice a week for about 45 minutes to 1 hour. For those who can't make two sessions in a week, they can opt for the 1 treatment that will last 90 minutes.

After the regular sessions, it is advisable to go back for follow up treatment. It should be every 2 weeks for the next 2 months and then once a month later on.

Aside from needles, most clinics use herbs in the form of masks, poultices and moisturizers. Before you use it, check with your doctor to make sure there is no allergic reaction to any forms of medication that you are taking.

After the first facial acupuncture treatment, you will usually seen an increased glow to one's complexion which the Chinese say an increased Qi or blood flow to the face. It becomes more open, the wrinkles start to disappear and the skin appears more toned.

In the 5th or 7th treatment, this becomes more evident as your face looks more relaxed as though you just came from a vacation.

The end result is that you will look and feel 5 to 15 years younger but of course this depends on how well the patient has taken care of themselves outside the confines of the clinic.

To sum things up, facial acupuncture can do for you. It can eliminate fine lines and reduces wrinkles, improve your overall facial color and add luster to the skin, relaxes tension in the face and furrows in the brow, brightens the eyes and reduce dark circles and puffiness, improve muscle tone for sagging skin, enhance your natural radiance in the skin and eyes, slow the aging process within, promotes overall health and well being as well as relaxes and revitalizes the entire body.

All you have to now is find a clinic that offers this service to customers so you will soon look radiant to other people.

Lower back pain plagues Americans to the extent that 80% will suffer from it at some time in their lives.   It is one of the most common reasons people visit the doctor.   For many, the problem is more than a passing incident; they need physiotherapy.

Physiotherapy of different types can be used to treat lower back pain.   Acupuncture is fast becoming an important method for the relief of such pain.   The doctor has the patient lie face-down and inserts the acupuncture needles across the back.   The doctor then finishes the procedure for lower back pain.   Pain relief after a series of treatments usually lasts months.

Massage is also used for lower back pain.   The massage used must be done by someone well-versed in the treatment of lower back pain.   A massage done by an untrained person may do more harm than good.

These methods are called passive therapies, or modalities.   They are done to the patient and not by the patient.   There are other modalities that are commonly used.   Heat and ice packs are a well-known form of passive physiotherapy.   They can be used separately, or they can be used alternately by a person who is suffering from acute lower back pain.

A transcutaneous electrical nerve stimulator (TENS) can be used as another modality for lower back pain.   The patient will feel the sensation of the stimulator instead of his pain.   If the TENS unit seems to work well for him, he will be sent home with one to use at his convenience.

Ultrasound is especially useful as a passive therapy for anyone with acute lower back pain.   It delivers heat deep into the muscles of the lower back.   This not only relieves pain.   It can also speed healing.

Back exercises may be assigned by a physiotherapist.   These exercises will help with lower back pain if one does them correctly and faithfully.   The only exception is if the back is in an acute condition requiring emergency care or surgery.

The exercises that will help with lower back pain the most will be assigned and supervised by a physiotherapist.   They may be done at home, but it will be necessary to follow instructions and check in frequently.

These exercises include ones for lower back pain that stretch or extend the back and ones that strengthen it.   One is an exercise where one lies prone and moves as if swimming.   This protects the back while giving the surrounding muscles a workout.

Lower back pain exercises called flexion exercises strengthen the midsection to provide support for the back.   If the lower back pain is reduced when one sits, these exercises are important. One is a knee-to-chest exercise.

Aerobic exercise such as walking is excellent for reducing and preventing lower back pain as well. Massage and acupuncture can be counted on to relieve pain for most patients. Exercises can make the back stronger to both relieve and prevent lower back pain. Any physiotherapy that can help relieve lower back pain will help millions of people.

www.ingramcontent.com/pod-product-compliance
Lightning Source LLC
Chambersburg PA
CBHW071253280526
45788CB00004B/1700